D1528148

Discover the Power
of
INTROVERSION

**What Most Introverts Are Never Told
and
Extraverts Learn
the Hard Way**

by

Cheryl N. W. Card

Published by the Type & Temperament Press

1

Table of Contents

Preface

Are you an Introvert or an Extravert? Do you prefer to focus your energy internally, on ideas, or do you prefer to focus your energy externally, on people, places, and things? We all do *both at times,* but we all have a natural bent toward one or the other.

Introverts and Extraverts are different. Both can be successful.
75% of the world are Extraverts. Are Introverts a downtrodden 25% minority? Not really. Lots of *"I's'"* are extremely successful in real-world terms. Two of the last four Presidents were Introverts, as are many corporation presidents, scientists, actors— every profession has successful Introverts. (Though some jobs require them to use their Extraverted side more often; others let them spend most of their time Introverting.)

But successful or not, Introverts are often misunderstood.

Even by themselves.

All their lives, Introverts have heard things like:

"Why have you got your door closed?"

"Come out of your room and meet our guests."

"Don't be shy."

"Why do I have to carry the whole conversation?"

"When someone asks you a question, just answer them. You don't have to spend all day thinking about it!"

"I wish you had lots of friends like your brother/ sister/ the kid next door."

"You spend so much time on one thing. You need more variety in your life."

Or sometimes, "You have such a beautiful smile. I wish you'd use it more often."

Extravert Parent, Introvert Child

With three Extraverts for every Introvert, there's a good chance that an Introvert will have at least one, and often two, Extraverted parents—who will expect the Introvert to "act like a good little Extravert." This may lead the Introvert to believe she or he is not OK, that something is wrong with them. The parents may even believe that. The child's uniquely Introverted needs may not get well met. (The reverse situation— an Extravert child raised by two Introverts—happens less often. It is also a problem, but less so because there are so many Extraverts out there as role models, and usually the Extravert child will naturally seek them out.)

The Gift of Introversion

Introverts are valuable, talented, effective people. The Introvert has gotten a "bum rap" for years in much of western culture. (In many eastern cultures, it is the Extraverts who must adjust.) The differences between *E's* and *I's* are important. Understanding them can help you understand yourself better, if you're an Introvert, and understand your "significant Introvert" better, if you're an Extravert.

This book will help you to

1) understand and *appreciate your strengths* if you're an Introvert;

2) provide you with *practical advice* to help you understand and relate to Introverts, if you're an Extravert; and

3) understand the importance of *developing* your Introverted side, if you're an Extravert.

In sum, this book will enable Introverts *and* Extraverts to value the gift of Introversion.

Dedication

This book is dedicated to my father,
Vernon Card, my first Introvert.

INTRODUCTION:

What *is* Introversion, Anyway?

1

Good News/Bad News

"And they were not ashamed."
The Book of Genesis

It's not considered "cool" to be an Introvert.

For one thing, 75% of the population in the United States is extraverted. So we Introverts are a minority.

And we get bad press— when we get any attention at all.

I just finished reading a mystery, **The Father Hunt,** by Rex Stout, featuring the great detective Nero Wolfe. Wolfe's assistant, Archie Goodwin, commented about a client, "One of the words she used was 'introvert,' which I would have supposed was moth-eaten for a girl just out of Smith."

Recently I looked up "Introvert" in the Reader's Guide to Periodical Literature. It said, "See Autism."

My father used to say he was an Introvert. He seemed clear about it but I can't say he sounded proud.

Many people consider "Introvert" to be synonymous with "shy." Introvert doesn't mean shy. Extraverts can be shy, and Introverts can be outgoing.

During a visit with my next-door neighbor, I mentioned that I was writing a book about Introversion. "I'm an Introvert," he said. "I know," I said, "me too. "First you have to decide it's OK to be one," said my neighbor. *"People don't want you to be."*

And that's the purpose of this book: to help us Introverts (and the Extraverts we know and love) understand that:

It's <u>OK</u> to be an Introvert.

It's more than OK. There is value to be appreciated and power to be discovered.

9

2

Are You An Introvert?

"My mistress is privacy. I'm having an affair with peace and quiet."
*Ben in **Broadway Bound** by Neil Simon*

The Swiss psychologist Carl G. Jung (1875-1961) recognized that we all have a preferred mode or attitude which we use to direct our mental functions. If I focus primarily on self and ask, "How does that relate to me?" then I am an Introvert. If, according to Jung, I focus on external things and ask, "How do I relate to that?", then I am an Extravert.

Another way of describing the difference between Introverts and Extraverts, or "*I' s*" and "*E' s*" as they can be referred to, is to describe the *source* of their energy:

I's "recharge" their batteries by being alone.

E's "recharge" their batteries by being with other people.

Extraverts embrace the outside world. They willingly give their attention to the people, objects and conditions around them. Introverts are often unaware of their surroundings and regard external claims on their attention as intrusive.

Jung believed that we have behavior preferences which are inborn, much like right- and left-handedness. Just as we can use either hand, we can choose to be in Introvert or Extravert mode. But we're naturally more comfortable with one than with the other.

Perhaps the following lists will help you decide whether your preference is for Introversion or Extraversion. No one has *all* the characteristics listed, and we all have some traits from *both* lists.

Which list is *more* descriptive of you?

Extraverts (E):	Introverts (I):
Talk	Listen
Outward	Inward
Enthusiastic	Intense
Sociable	Private
Confident	Questioning
Spend energy	Save energy
Many friends	A few friends
Talk, then think	Think, then maybe talk
Act, then think	Think, then maybe act
Initiate	Consider
Auditory	Visual
Involvement	Detachment
Results-oriented	Idea-oriented
Propagate/expend	Conserve/consolidate
Broad interests/ generalist	Depth of interest/ specialist
Doesn't understand life 'til lived it	Won't live life 'til understands it

The Four Mental Functions

Carl Jung also identified four mental functions. We all have two *perceiving or information-gathering* functions:

Sensing (S) (for tangible things)

Intuition (N) (for abstract possibilities).

In addition, we all have two *judging or organizing* functions:

Thinking (T) (decides logically or objectively)

Feeling (F) (decides based on values or subjectively).

The letters are used by the Myers-Briggs Type Indicator.®* The MBTI®* also identifies whether people prefer to be in Judging (J) or Perceiving (P) mode when dealing with the external world. (With Judging people, we most often hear their judgments; with Perceiving people, we most often hear their perceptions.)

Another definition of Introvert deals with how one *uses* these mental functions. The function we use most, our "right hand" so to speak, is our Dominant function. Our second most preferred function is called our Auxiliary. Extraverts use their Dominant (best) function to deal with the external world. Introverts use their Dominant (best) function inside and use their Auxiliary (second-best) to deal with the outside world.

Introverts and Extraverts differ in what they present to the world. Extraverts show the world what is most important to them. Introverts keep what is most important inside. If Introverts seem difficult to know, that is why. They are not always what they seem.

*Myers-Briggs Type Indicator® and MBTI® are registered trademarks of Consulting Psychologists Press, Palo Alto, CA.

A PART OF
AND
APART FROM

3

One of Life's Big Secrets

Before you can say "I love you," you have to be able to say " I."

Ayn Rand

A secret well kept, from Introverts and Extraverts alike, is:

> *There is a very important part of all Extraverts that is Introverted!*

Moreover, *if Extraverts don't get in touch with their Introvert side*, they will not be utilizing an important mental capacity.

The second most important mental function of Extraverts is used in Introvert mode. Without that, Extraverts are not as powerful as they might be. In fact, without utilizing their Introvert side, Extraverts will be operating minus two or even three of their four basic functions!

Our four mental functions are used in alternate modes: If a person's dominant function is Extraverted, his or her auxiliary is Introverted. The Extravert's fourth or "inferior" function is also Introverted. If a person's Dominant is Introverted, then his or her Auxiliary and Inferior (second and fourth) functions are Extraverted.

There is disagreement about the use of the third function. Some believe balance is achieved by alternating mode of use, in which case the third function would be used in the same mode as the Dominant. Others believe balance is achieved by using the Dominant in one mode and the other three functions in the other mode.

In any case, we cannot be *whole* without using both our Extravert and Introvert parts.

4

Life Isn't Fair to Introverts

"They mean well but they are so social they are nearly hive- minded. They cannot understand that one might wish to be without company."

Wintermoon in
Winds of Change by
Mercedes Lackey

It is possible for Extraverts to live their entire lives and never become acquainted with their Introvert mode. But Introverts *must* Extravert in order to function in society.

You've heard of hermits (I'm sure it's no coincidence

that I've never met one); however, most of us grow up living with others. Children are thrust into school, often after already being in pre-school and day care. Adolescents have to use Extravert mode to accomplish the task of finding their place in the world. Often it's extremely difficult for Introverts—of any age— to find "alone time."

I remember often "bowing out" of office get-togethers, even occasionally Christmas parties. At the time, I didn't know exactly why — I just knew I didn't want to go. Sometimes I made excuses, but they masked the real meaning: to go just felt overwhelming. I simply needed to be alone for some "down-time." However, not understanding *why*, I felt totally inadequate; moreover, not even the people closest to me (those I thought really "knew" me) understood. So in addition to feeling like there was something *wrong* with me, I felt guilty .

Because I now understand my Introversion, *I am able to accept myself.* If I've "used up" my energy for "Extraverting" and need time alone to "recharge," I no longer make excuses. I simply tell the truth. And the result is that I no longer think there's something wrong with me or feel guilty because I can't live up to someone else's expectation. But the journey has been a very long and frustrating one.

5

Differences in Brain Chemistry

"I gotta hide someplace to find myself again."
Roger Miller in Big River

One reason why Introverts seek peace and quiet and privacy more than Extraverts may be found in a difference in the normal level of brain activity.

In Larry Morris's book *Extraversion and Introversion,* he examines three decades of research by Hans Eysenck which led to the conclusion that "Introverts typically have higher levels of cortical arousal compared with Extraverts." Similar findings were reported by Martha A. Wilson and Marlin L. Languis in a recent *Journal of Psychological Type.**

Seeking to balance this discrepancy, Introverts tend to avoid additional stimulation (provided by the external world), while Extraverts tend to seek additional stimulation and arousal.

*"Differences in Brain Electrical Activity Patterns between Introverted and Extraverted Adults," Wilson & Languis, JPT Vol 18, 1989.

Other research suggests that it is not simply the overall degree of arousal that is responsible for a physiological difference between Introverts and Extraverts but rather differences regarding attention spans, depth of emotions, and possibly even responses to visual versus auditory stimuli.

Whatever scientists will find to be the exact nature, it is clear that *there are physiological differences between E's and I's.*

For Introverts, the opposite of an uncomfortable state of arousal is a peaceful centeredness which with practice can be achieved in the presence of company and commotion, but is more easily reached alone.

In my own life in the past few years I have observed more clearly the tension I experience from using my Extravert "left hand." I used to think I just got a lot of tension headaches at work. Now, much as I love teaching about personality type, it's always a relief to be alone again. I am acutely aware of the blessed process of "settling down."

THE VALUE OF INTROVERSION

6

The Introvert/ Archetype Connection

"Until we become thoroughly aware of the inad-equacy of our extraverted state and of its insufficiency in regard to our deeper spiritual needs, we shall not achieve even a measure of individuation, through which a wider and more mature personality emerges."
Stephen A. Hoeller, **The Gnostic Jung**

Introverts need to know that although, or perhaps because, they are not in the mainstream, they have unique value.

Introverts seem to have a closer connection with the collective unconscious that stores human progress known as *archetypes*. Archetypes, according to Carol S. Pearson in *Awakening The Heroes Within**, can be used by everyone as inner guides; they are deep, eternal, primal images reflected in art, literature, myth, and religion. They can link our longing and pain with those who have come before, teaching us how to connect to the great and timeless cycles of the natural and spiritual worlds. It is my belief that Introverts, some more than others and some more consciously than others, tap more frequently and more easily into this rich reservoir.

This mysterious "understanding," independent of external opinions and events, can serve as a grounding force in the world. For Extraverts, the external world IS reality. For Introverts, *their perception* of the external world is what matters. That perception, formed by things inside them, goes deep.

I have a friend who for years has kept her brightest light under a bushel. Feeling anxiety and even shame over revealing her deepest self, she is slowly beginning to invite her creativity to show itself in the form of crafts and music. It is common for her to *make a connection* between extremely diverse things. For example, she may see the bark on a particular tree as of the same "essence" as the jazz saxophone music of John Coltrane, as a group of pre-abstract Mondrian

* Carol S. Pearson, "Awakening the Heroes Within,"pg. 2 HarperSanFrancisco 1991

paintings, and as the line (from "Among School Children") by Yeats "can't tell the dancers from the dance." It is, however, uncommon for her, as an Introvert, to share this knowledge from her Introverted iNtuition.

A dominant Introverted Sensor might have a similar— but very different— experience. The wealth of images stored by dominant Sensing is rich in detail, and is experience-based: pictures (sounds, tastes, smells, sensations) perceived in the past, in a similar situation, that come flooding back to allow one to understand a new situation. The bottom line may warn the Sensor away from the new idea, or relate it positively to experience so that it is deemed "OK." But it can be felt as just a "knowing," based on experience.

If one's dominant function is an Introverted *deciding* function (Thinking or Feeling) rather than a perceptive one (Sensing or iNtuition), the result may well be an unshakeable decision, which the Introvert may or may not want to bother defending verbally— but may be most unwilling to change without significant additional information. This is especially true of Feelers, whose decision criteria are subjective and personal, as opposed to Thinkers' logical approach. Input that would logically change the situation, will, if proven true, generally change the Thinker's mind.

Type, as part of the Ego, will filter the appeal of different archetypes at different times and affect how and whether we connect with them.* Different types may relate more readily to some archetypes than to others.

Whatever one's preferred function (Sensing, iNtuition, Thinking or Feeling), everyone has and can use iNtuition. Whether you prefer Introverted iNtuition or Extraverted iNtuition, the iNtuitive function connects at some level with the wellsprings of the unconscious. Those who prefer to Introvert their iNtuition (NJs or SPs, in MBTI terms), may find meditation especially useful in accessing it. Those who prefer to Introvert Sensing (SJs and NPs) may find meditation useful in accessing practical experiential input, stored away in their mental depths.

We all need more of this Introverted insight to deal with the pace and multitude of options facing us in today's world. For the first half of my life I tried to make choices by analyzing things, solving problems, actively figuring out what to do. Several years ago, I realized that it's usually easier to simply *allow myself to know.* Of course, I still collect external data, talk things over with others, and make lists of "pro's" and "con's." But after doing all of this "figuring," I become *still* and trust that the decision will come to me, rather like a bubble rising to the surface.

*"Type & Archetype," Carol S. Pearson, Type & Temperament, Inc.1994

Letting yourself "know" can be done by deliberately sitting quietly and opening the mind, a form of meditation. Or it can be done by not trying to decide right away, letting the issue "process"—simply waiting.

I believe that accessing this "internal" wisdom is a nearly pure form of "Introvert processing." I also believe that this wisdom often comes from a higher power, from a timeless reservoir of images and energy. A possible course of action is of the same "essence" as (i.e., somehow "fits") a developing part of you, and you *know* that, just as my friend *knew* about certain connections. (The difficulty of "figuring out" is that there seems to be no end to the process, as one can often build a case for each side.) Going inside to make a decision automatically filters out what is irrelevant and brings focus and clarity. Of course, you can overdo this. The Introvert must balance this process of knowing from within with some amount of Extraverting, in order to connect with reality.

We desperately need visions to guide us personally and in my view, as a society. For example, Woodrow Wilson *knew* that the world needed an international governing body. His Introversion may have kept him from realizing this "dream" at the time. But the *idea* eventually moved us along.

Too often, perhaps because Introverts aren't as verbal

as Extraverts, or as well connected with the outside world, the insights and wisdom of Introverts are not recognized. We may have to *wait* to hear from Introverts. But their input is usually well worth waiting for!

7

Creating Positive Self-Image "The *I's* Have It..."

"...the Introverts' advantages need to be pointed out — not only to the Extraverts but sometimes even to the Introverts themselves — for the best-adjusted people are the 'psychologically patriotic,' who are glad to be what they are."
Isabel Briggs Myers with Peter B. Myers,
Gifts Differing

When my daughter, having taken the Myers-Briggs Type Indicator at age 12, understood that she was an Introvert and that Introverts have special value, it made an enormous difference in how she felt about herself. She had always felt *different* from other children. Now she could perceive that difference in a way that made her feel *good* about herself rather than feeling that something was wrong with her.

As mentioned previously, in the United States we are about 75% Extraverts and 25% Introverts. And as my neighbor indicated, being an Introvert means not being in the mainstream.

I have another Introvert friend who is an engineer, retired from a large corporation. After he read a draft of this book, he made me promise to address the "frustration and pain" involved in being an Introvert.

He was aware that he was an Introvert but that had not always been the case. He'd grown up in a family where he was encouraged to be "successful." After college, he found a respectable sales position, trying hard to work his way "up the ladder." Success was defined by those around him as more clients and higher commissions. He knew he was intelligent and hard-working, but somehow he never "succeeded" in the prescribed way. For years he agonized over what was wrong with him, trying to analyze his "failure."

Now he believes that he should have taken another path, perhaps choosing an academic career, or working in corporate research and development. He had made a common mistake: not honoring his Introvert preference and *using* it rather than fighting it, trying for years to be something he was not. He feels regret, and understandably, a certain amount of anger. Perhaps the world got a good salesman —but lost a great creative mind.

An interesting — and profound— question to ask is: How many creative minds are lost because they are not supported and honored?

THE CHALLENGE
OF
INTROVERT
CHILDREN

8

A Room of One's Own

(or Introvert Kids at Home)

*"It's like an acorn going through excruci-
ating agony for becoming an oak, or a
flower feeling ashamed for blossoming."*

Healing the Shame that Binds You, *by
John Bradshaw*

Some observers believe that babies who cuddle in their blankets and sleep a lot are Introverts, and babies who wiggle off covers and demand a lot of attention are Extraverts. (Of course Introverts could be collicky and Extraverts could be tired !)

Certainly a difference can be observed in young children, some of whom when arriving at a playground stand back to "check things out," while others jump right in. Some children are stressed by an absence of playmates and external stimuli; other children are stressed by too much interaction.

Some interesting observations were made by a friend of mine who for years taught kindergarten and is now a Myers-Briggs practitioner. She remembers what she would now identify as Introvert/Extravert differences in pre-school children whom she was testing. She noticed that some children, Introverts no doubt, became upset when a great deal of interaction was demanded in testing, either with the examiner or with other children. On the other hand, children whom she would now identify as Extraverts, were frustrated when she would silently observe their activities. She vividly remembers one child who walked over, stared up into her face, burst into tears, and called to his mother, "She won't talk to me!"

We've all heard stories about times when left-handed children were not allowed to be left-handed!(Some even had an arm tied down by a well-meaning teacher.) Too many children have had similar experiences with psychological preferences.

Parents and teachers may try to make Extraverts out of Introverts and Introverts out of Extraverts. An Introvert child of Extravert parents may be told to "speak up," "get involved," and "raise your hand" in school. He or she may be criticized for wanting to sit and read when " there are all those opportunities out there!" The Extravert child of Introvert parents may be considered hyperactive and disruptive, perhaps even be severely disciplined for excessive talking and touching. These children are not being contrary. They are simply being true to themselves.

Introvert children with preference for "feeling" rather than "thinking" may be more comfortable with a companion. But for the most part, Introverts are their own best friends. They may enjoy being alone and sometimes may feel lonely in groups. Being asked to "come out and play" means coming out from inside themselves, which demands a lot of effort. Extraverts need to remember that this process drains energy from Introverts, even when they are small children.

Helpful Hints for Parenting

For Extravert parents of Introvert children:
(or Introvert parents of Introvert children):

Here are some suggestions for supporting Introvert children:

> Wait to ask about their experiences until they have processed and recharged and are ready to tell you.
>
> Help them find courteous ways to find the time they need away from people.
>
> Discuss IN PRIVATE any need for changes in behavior.
>
> Incorporate breaks from socializing into family schedules.
>
> Recognize that inadequate "alone" time is a reason for tantrums, irritability, aggression, and other behavior problems, with siblings as well as with other children.
>
> Find ways to honor the Introvert's need for physical space, from not sitting too close, to a room of his or her own.

Don't press them to be more outgoing than they can handle. One or two close friends is probably enough.

Help them create "scripts" for saying "no" to their Extravert friends when they need to.

Help the Introvert avoid interruptions, which rob energy.

Don't demand immediate responses. Introverts need processing time.

Respect the need for privacy.

With a little rephrasing, you can also use the foregoing ideas :

To help Extraverts develop their Introvert side for a healthy, balanced life.

To help Introvert parents take care of themselves.

To nurture our inner child, especially if our Introversion was not supported when we were children.

To deal with any personal relationships with Introverts.

Likewise Introverts have a responsibility to honor Extraversion. Following are some thoughts about that.

For Introvert parents of Extravert children:
(or Extravert parents of Extravert children):

Here are some suggestions for supporting your Extravert child.

Realize that, unlike Introverts, Extraverts tend to think by talking, *not before* talking, and give them opportunities to do this. *Remember*: What they say will probably not be their final word on the subject.

Help them find acceptable opportunities to touch things, talk with people, and interact in general. That may not be how you process but that's how they process.

Emphasize taking turns — even if they have to practice patience waiting for an Introvert friend to take advantage of the opportunity!

Help them to learn how to respond to signals from other people that they have talked enough; teach them skills to limit themselves.

Find non-damaging ways children can handle things in stores while helping sales personnel understand that you are aware of their concern.

While Introverts study better alone, Extraverts may need to study with friends or at least discuss what they're learning with a parent.

And, hard as it may be for us Introverts to believe, some people do find it more comfortable (and even effective) to study with the TV or radio on!

Awareness of one another's needs as well as of one another's "gifts differing" makes us all stronger, happier, and more productive.

9

"Introverts Know the Answer, Just Let Them Reflect On It."
(or Introvert Kids at School)

Extraverts and Introverts have different needs in the classroom. Making a classroom challenging and comfortable for all the different personality types and temperaments seems to be an impossible task. (That has never stopped good teachers from doing it!) Often the most workable solution is to include a variety of approaches.

Introvert students are usually fairly comfortable with the traditional classroom and with lecture-style presentations. The quiet activities involved in learning — reading, writing, homework, test-taking — don't inherently cause them discomfort. Being alone while they learn allows Introverts the process time they need.

Extraverts prefer interactive learning. They need to get up and move. Because their thinking process is verbalized, they need to discuss what they're learning. They are eager for hands-on experience. They like group projects, will volunteer, and will contribute to discussion "off the top of their head." Not so the Introverts.

Introverts want to think over what is being presented. If they are to participate in discussion or make a presentation themselves, they will want time (minutes, if not days) to complete their mental processing, prepare, and rehearse, in their heads if not in actuality.

During this "process time," which Extraverts sometime perceive as hesitation or slowness, Introverts are searching inside for something to which to attach the new information. They often prefer to be given the theory first and then hang specifics on it, something like decorating a Christmas tree. Extraverts want the action first before trying to understand the theory.

It is important for teachers to understand this difference among their students as well as to understand their own preference. An Introvert teacher may consider Extravert students undisciplined. An Extravert teacher may not understand the needs of the Introvert.

Especially when class participation counts for a grade, it is helpful for teachers to give the Introverts time— time to get acquainted with other students as well as time to think. Announcing topics beforehand gives Introverts the chance to mull things over. Opportunities for one-on-one discussion and individual projects are helpful. Dividing a class into smaller groups for discussion often makes Introverts more comfortable.

The typical difference in behavior between Extraverts and Introverts is forever imprinted on my mind by an experience I had teaching the Myers-Briggs Type Indicator to a high school drama class. We had just completed an exercise where Introverts and Extraverts say what they like and dislike about Introversion and Extraversion. After making sure both groups had their say on each topic, the teacher and I opened the floor for discussion.

Seated where they had been for the group work, Extraverts were on one side of the room and Introverts on the other. Picture this:

The Extraverts, on my left, were barely able to remain seated. They squirmed and stretched upward to get my attention. All hands were in the air at about a 45 degree angle, waving sideways and up and down. They could barely wait for a turn to speak. Their energy clamored. Breathing was irregular. Their eye contact with me was intense as they willed me to call on them.

On my right, the Introverts were seated quietly. They had no less interest, but they had no urge to jump out of their seats. They, too, shared a common posture. But their intensity was displayed by stillness. Arms were folded, or chins were thoughtfully on hands, or pens were toyed with. Some eyes were down, some on me, some on the Extraverts.

The teacher and I exchanged an understanding glance, and I began calling on students. I called on an Extravert first, to get some group relief and give the Introverts time to process.

10

"I'm Just Not a Party Person"
(or Introverts at College)

As the Introvert child grows into young adulthood and enters college, he or she faces a host of complex issues. The majority of students are Extraverts. They talk. Several may talk at once. No one really listens. Except maybe Introverts.

"Partying," "hanging out" and talking until dawn seem to be the thing. (If all this sounds uninteresting to you, you may be an Introvert.)

Introverts *do* need to socialize. But they'd like it to be worth the effort. It's important to remember: for Introverts the discomfort of being in "Extravert mode" is what anyone would experience if asked to write with the less preferred hand.

Introverts often choose to socialize by participating in a project where the purpose is foremost and social-izing occurs along the way. They may enjoy study groups — provided they also have opportunities to study alone.

There's no question that college-bound Introverts need to be aware they'll have to work harder at getting established socially. For one thing, it's obviously difficult for Introverts to find each other. Choosing to room alone may help: it provides "space" and relief from the outside world. Or it may make things more difficult because there is no built-in companion.

It is important for Introverts to simply be aware of these issues and to remember that there are others (probably 25% of the student body) who feel the same way. (And when getting established at college, even the Extraverts may be uncomfortable.) It is important for Introverts to stretch but stay true to themselves.

An Introvert Advantage

Introverts tend to be good students, and this is partly because they often enjoy reading more than Extraverts; moreover, they tend to be more comfortable "putting things in writing. " Writing allows Introverts to finish arranging their ideas using their dominant, Introverted function before "going public."

In a sense the steps in the process of writing are reversed for the two types. For Introverts it is *Think, Write, Talk.* For Extraverts it is *Talk, Write, Think..*

In getting started, to find inspiration or to "brainstorm," Extraverts will consider what they and others have already said on the subject as well as their own broad experience. Introverts may "brainstorm" internally first, consulting a different kind of personal experience. They are more apt to consider what they have read and how all of this relates to their internal framework. (Introverts need to avoid thinking deeply for *too* long before moving to the task at hand, so they don't make things overly complex.)

When the actual writing phase begins, Introverts are usually most comfortable being by themselves in order to arrange their ideas. Extraverts, on the other hand, must make an effort to work by themselves; they are always more tolerant of interruptions. (My Extravert friends have told me they can write more easily if they approach the first draft as if they are simply "talking" through their ideas.)

In rewriting, the two preferences need to include what they have not already, naturally done. *I's* need to add information from experiences — theirs and others'. Introverts often need reality checks. They need to seek input and/or feedback from others before considering a project finished. Introverts need to

45

be sure that what makes sense to them also makes sense to others.

E's usually need to do some serious thinking before a work is finished, consulting their Introvert side to combine ideas in their own framework. They, too, should seek feedback from others, perhaps including some Introverts. Extraverts often need to focus on a few points and add depth, while Introverts may need to add breadth.

Both types need to work towards condensing or "tightening" as they re-write, though for different reasons. *E's* often need to omit unnecessary words and paragraphs. *I's* may need to remove some complexities.

MAKING GOOD DECISIONS IN THE REAL WORLD

11

Career Considerations for Introverts

"The greatest man I never knew. . .
The greatest words I never heard."

Song by Reba McEntire

In *Gifts Differing*, Myers and Myers describe Extraverts as "the civilizing genius, the people of action and practical achievement." Introverts are described as "the cultural genius, the people of ideas and abstract invention."

Introverts need Extraverts (and their own Extravert capability) for information from the real world. Extraverts need Introverts (and their own Introvert capability) for ideas. Without one another, Introverts may be overly intellectual and often unrealistic; Extraverts may be prone to be driven by external conditions and or other people.

Introverts usually prefer jobs where they work alone or with a few people, where they can utilize their powers of concentration, reflect before acting or taking a position, read, and put things in writing. They are good with ideas and concepts and comfortable handling lengthy, complex projects. They may resist taking time for social niceties and often have difficulty remembering names.

Extraverts, on the other hand, usually prefer a work environment with lots of people, where there is variety and situations which involve talking through ideas. They are curious about all aspects of the organization and often enjoy talking on the phone. Impatient with lengthy, slow-moving projects, they like action. They are natural with "public relations;"

their out-going nature often puts people at ease.

Occupations often preferred by Extraverts include marketing, sales, public relations, reception, performing, education, religion.

Occupations often preferred by Introverts include secretary, librarian, scientist, lawyer, researcher, physician, priest/minister, editor, pharmacist, engineer, computer programmer.

It is important to remember, however, that a person of either preference can be successful in any position, depending upon strength of preference, versatility, age, motivation, life circumstance, and simply the mix of job and individual.

12

Office Politics: "Quiet Please, Out to Lunch"

You may notice Introverts seeking peace and quiet during lunchtime. If they stay in, *I's* may shut their office door and eat alone. If they lunch with company, it's more apt to be with one other person than with a large group. Or if they shop or exercise during lunch, they will probably do so alone. In contrast, Extraverts will most likely eat, shop or exercise in groups. Each is re-charging in his or her own way.

There are, of course, exceptions. Since lunch is break time, if an Introvert works alone, he or she may choose to socialize at meal time. Or if an Extravert works constantly with people, he or she may need some time alone.

You will often find Introverts reading while eating, preferring the undemanding company of a book. I am fiercely protective of this private practice. (I have developed incredible skill at eating with one hand so I can hold a book in the other!)

Things that Extraverts probably enjoy more than Introverts, indeed that I's may find irritating and invasive, include:

- Walkmen® (Why walk if not to enjoy peace and quiet?)
- car phones (The car may be the only place l can be alone!)
- cordless phones (Phones should be kept in their place.)
- Muzak® — in elevators; and especially while waiting on the phone.

People who make Introverts feel uncomfortable, if not angry, include:
- "greeters"— effusively cheerful people who expect a response
- "familiars" (What gives you the right to call me by my first name?)
- telemarketers — another invasion of privacy

A Workable Work Environment
I once had the pleasure of working in a small, all-Introvert office. At the time I was the single parent of

three young children, and work in that quiet, orderly setting was an incredibly soothing experience. Socializing occurred regularly but briefly and infrequently during the day. Socializing with clients for the most part took place on trips. We were rarely interrupted with phone calls. Everyone ate lunch at his desk unless there were business appointments. On Fridays we went out to lunch together, usually returning in the hour time slot.

Internal communication was smooth and clear and took place as necessary. The business was focused and prosperous.

That experience was probably unique. In most businesses, efforts must be made for Introverts *and* Extraverts to work together in order to take advantage of their different strengths, needs, and interests.

Suggestions to help this process include:

- Include opportunities for discussion for the Extraverts
- Include opportunities to put things in writing for the Introverts
- Give Introverts adequate time for reflection
- Honor the Introverts' need for unbroken concentration and freedom from interruption.

BUILDING
SATISFYING
RELATIONSHIPS

13

Potential Extravert/ Introvert Conflict

"Avoid loud & aggressive persons, they are vexatious to the spirit."

Desiderata

Extraverts may perceive Introverts to be unresponsive. Introverts may see Extraverts as shallow.

In workshop groups, asked what they dislike about Introverts, Extraverts identified the following:
- It's difficult to start up conversation
- They're too serious
- They're " party poopers"
- You don't know where you stand because they don't "emote"
- They're slow; they slow down the process
- They're a mystery

Asked what they like about Introverts, Extraverts responded:
- They're considerate
- They're good listeners
- They have great ideas

What Introverts liked about Extraverts was:

- They take responsibility for talking
- They volunteer
- They're good at parties and holidays
- They're entertaining

What Introverts didn't like about Extraverts was:

- They're noisy and tiring
- They interrupt
- They assume everybody wants to participate
- They assume we (Introverts) are or should be like them

14

Honoring the Differences

"I know a little bit about practically everything."
An Extravert
"I guess that means I know almost everything
about practically nothing."
An Introvert

Prince Charles and Princess Diana illustrate the classic Introvert-Extravert conflict with couples. She likes nightclubs and lots of activity. He needs time for solitary contemplation. They struggled unsuccessfully to find a way to live together yet meet their respective needs. Neither is wrong. Each had the potential of being a great asset to the other. There are surely other personality differences (as well as other problems) between Charles and Diana but certainly the E-I difference is a major one.

I know couples whose Myers-Briggs Type Indicator letters are all the same except for E and I. They generally get along well, but the Introvert almost always says that his or her partner had *to learn* to respect the Introvert's need for time alone. Extraverts often don't understand this need. They take it personally and feel rejected. (This reaction occurs among friends as well as with couples.)

Allowance always has to be made for different styles. Extraverts process externally and want to talk a lot. Introverts process internally and often don't talk until they've reached a conclusion. Extraverts tend to externalize problems, hence may blame the Introvert. Introverts tend to internalize things, hence may blame themselves. Introverts need to suspend their urge to go inside long enough to listen, even if they've heard this before. (What can be taken in that might be new?)

Extraverts need to be still and to listen when the Introvert does talk. It may seem like too little, too late. But remember that the bit of energy revealed is the tip of an iceberg — perhaps more accurately, the tip of a bonfire. Extraverts need to be patient and not overwhelm their Introvert partner with demands to *share*, because that only makes the Introvert withdraw further. It's helpful if Introverts learn that it's OK to share incomplete thoughts and feelings, perhaps identifying them as such.

By tempering the energy of their dominant preference with respect for another's different gifts, partners
in a relationship can complement one another. When
opposites attract, it's for a reason. Extraverts may
encourage Introverts to go out more, make more
friends, participate in more activities. Introverts can
encourage Extraverts to take more time for themselves. If both partners genuinely respect each
other's differences, a healthy, creative balance can
be achieved.

The wonderful bonus from this technique is that
each person becomes more powerful not only by
association with the other's talents but because *in
honoring the other's preferences, one is also honoring and therefore strengthening those parts of one's
self.* Each partner is further developing his or her own
personality by strengthening the auxiliary function,
and the less frequently used attitude, be it Introversion or Extraversion.

CONTRIBUTIONS OF INTROVERTS TO CIVILIZATION

15

The Value of Their Leadership

"Be still and know..."
Psalm 46: 10

Behind every quantum step taken by humankind, I suspect there is an Introvert process at work, tapping into the unconscious, individual and collective, going *in and out:* observing the external world, going inside to ponder it, coming back out with an idea to offer. The same process that connects an individual with the knowledge of the needs of his or her archetype connects groups of people with the mythology, history, needs and aspirations of their culture.

One of the most profound historical examples of the influence of an Introvert is the leadership of Abraham Lincoln. Lincoln has been described as aloof, brooding, and inaccessible despite efforts at conviviality; introspective, tormented, deep—adjectives frequently applied to the Introvert personality. His soul-searching included ideas from Scripture, Shakespeare, dreams, and his personal history. We find themes of death, fatherhood, madness, and guilt mingled with freedom, martyrdom, rebirth and immortality.

In Lincoln's words, "there has fallen upon me a task such as did not rest even upon the father of this country..." The convergence of history and Lincoln's personality was so powerful that people still devote their entire lives to studying him. We often turn to his speeches and writings for guidance. People in other countries study him to understand America better. One can barely imagine this period in American history without Abraham Lincoln.

16

The Gift of Their Creativity

Think of the great scholars, philosophers, writers, poets, composers, and artists. A few, for example Socrates, "thought out loud." But most retired to seclusion to read, to reflect, to write, to experience their pain or to assimilate their joy. The insights and the associations they offer humankind come from places deep inside.

The Introvert process can be profoundly creative.

This does not mean that *only* Introverts are creative or that *all* Introverts are creative. Some Introverts don't know they can be creative; some Extraverts certainly use their Introvert function to generate ideas. (I don't include here the kind of creativity involved in resourceful organization of existing things.) And I am aware that a "group energy" often operates, for example, in the process of brainstorming. However, (as stated earlier), I believe that people *go inside* for ideas—particularly those who Introvert their iNtuition. They may be stimulated or inspired by external conditions. And of course the worldliness and resourcefulness of the Extraverted functions are essential in expressing, developing, and managing these new ideas.

Creativity seems to involve a breakthrough by an unconscious process. Sometimes what emerges is a specific idea, perhaps already associated with words or numbers. Sometimes it is a clear image or picture. Other times it is only a vague idea or shifting image that requires more thought and interpretation.

Again we see the Introvert's natural process of "in and out;" something happens in the external world, one takes it inside, and over time, something new emerges which can be shared with the world.

17

Famous Introverts

As you identify your preference for Introversion or Extraversion, you may be interested in the company you keep. Famous Introverts probably include St. Francis of Assisi, George Washington, Henry Ford, Thomas Edison, Sigmund Freud, Carl Jung, Joan of Arc, Albert Einstein, Calvin Coolidge, Herbert Hoover, and Abraham Lincoln.

Famous living Introverts probably include Richard Nixon, Katharine Hepburn, Red Adair, Nancy Reagan, Jimmy Carter, Jacqueline Onassis, and Prince Charles.

Famous Introvert characters may include Radar of M.A.S.H., Linus and Charlie Brown from *Peanuts*, Ashley Wilkes in *Gone With the Wind*, Perry Mason, Nero Wolfe, Huckleberry Finn, Hamlet, Macbeth, and the Phantom of the Opera.

Famous Extraverts might include John Kennedy, Will Rogers, Martin Luther King, Jr., Theodore and Franklin D. Roosevelt; Generals Patton and

Eisenhower; Ronald Reagan, and "Fergie," the Duchess of York.

Famous Extravert characters might include Edith Bunker, Lucy, Scarlett O'Hara, Tom Sawyer, Tevye from *Fiddler on the Roof*, Dolly Levi of *Matchmaker*, Puck and Falstaff.

Notice that the source of the fame and power of these personalities relates to their preference for Introversion or Extraversion. Extraverts are noteworthy because of how they connect with the external world. Introverts influence us because of their connection with internal forces.

WHAT IS
THIS THING
CALLED
PSYCHOLOGICAL
TYPE?

18

The Myers Briggs Type Indicator

One place where you do find the word *Introvert* used, and used a lot, is in the "Type Community," that is, among people who study psychological type, and most of whom administer the Myers-Briggs Type Indicator® (MBTI®), an instrument of *normal* psychology.

Based on the work of Carl Jung and developed by Isabel Briggs Myers, the Indicator measures individual preferences on four scales, one being *Introvert-Extravert*. The others deal with the mental functions of (1) *perceiving* and (2) *organizing* or *deciding*, as discussed briefly in an earlier chapter.

The two perceiving functions are Sensing and iNtuition. If I prefer sensing (*S*), I use my five senses to perceive facts and realities. I am practical. If I prefer iNtuition (*N*), I perceive possibilities with my "sixth" sense. I am imaginative. (75% of us are Sensors and 25% iNtuitives.)

The two organizing or judging functions are Thinking and Feeling. If I am a Thinker, I evaluate information based on logic and consequences. *T's* are impartial and can seem distant. If I am a Feeler, I evaluate information based on my values, what seems "good." *F's* are sympathetic and value harmony. (Overall we are 50% Thinkers and 50% Feelers. However, men are 60% Thinkers and 40% Feelers; and women are 60% Feelers and 40% Thinkers.)

The Myers-Briggs Type Indicator includes a fourth scale which describes how one deals with the external world: Do I prefer to use my Perceptive function or my Judging function? *P's* like to seek more information, to keep their options open, to "go with the flow." Whereas *J's* like to have things settled, decided, planned, put in place. (Overall, we are about 50% *J's* and *50% P's*, perhaps slightly more *J's*.)

The combinations of these four pairs of preferences yield sixteen personality types. Most people find that the Myers-Briggs Type Indicator describes them quite well.

Think of it this way: Each of us is the leader (director, coach, manager) of a group (cast, team, staff) of eight: E, I, S, N, T, F, J and P (Extraversion, Introversion, Sensing, iNtuition, Thinking, Feeling, Judging, & Perceiving). We decide when it is appropriate for each player to operate and to what extent. We are influenced by inborn preferences as well as life experience. Moreover, at different stages of life, we will probably make different choices.

19

Introverted and Extraverted Functions

We can use the four functions just described in either Introvert or Extravert mode. Which types do which and the order of influence of the functions is a subject too broad for this book. For our purposes here, we will simply examine how the functions differ when focused on the *internal* versus the *external* world.

People who extravert their judging function will share conclusions and move the conversation toward closure. Perceptive types may either welcome or resent this pressure to decide. Extraverted *J's* may become quiet when it comes to sharing information. This happens because their Perceptive function is used in Introvert mode, for psychological balance. Extraverted *J's* who are Thinking types can seem overly argumentative with their opinions. They are more tentative with new information and may need time alone to process it. Extraverted Feelers can seem too certain they know the right thing for someone (else) to do.

People who extravert or display their perceptive function like to open up conversations and explore. They do express judgments but tend to do so guardedly or hypothetically. They may need to be alone to arrive at a conclusion, since their preferred Judging function is normally used in Introvert mode. (Even if they are Extraverts.)

People who introvert Sensing are aware of tangible things as they pertain to self. They tend to have strong preferences about food, textures, colors, music, etc. They may be more aware than other types of bodily sensations.

People who extravert Sensing may collect unlimited detailed information about the lives of other people and things. They may have great interest in material possessions or in their surroundings.

People who introvert iNtuition like to be off by themselves to consider complex things, and like to do it on paper.

I am a dominant introverted iNtuitive and strongly resent intrusions on my "daydreaming." Obviously, though, I can't do that all the time. I remind myself of this when I have to prepare for a class, write a report, or attend to administrative details or children, not to mention to remember where I parked my car!

People who extravert iNtuition have a lot of ideas about what's going on around them (and in the larger world) and like to talk about all these possibilities.

Introverted Feelers are tuned in to how they feel about things but do not expect others to feel the same way. Their energy connects in some sense, with the archetypes of humanity and with powerful creative insights. In comparison with these great forces, they can sometimes feel inadequate.

Extraverted Feelers relate to the feelings of others, sometimes to an extreme. They are perplexed if others don't value the same things they do. Introverts who extravert feeling (not the dominant function) may be mistaken for Extraverts because they connect with people and have such empathy. (Ironically they may sometimes be more acutely aware of people in general than of loved ones.)

Introverted Thinkers look at their own life with the utmost of logic and are usually not very aware of their feelings.

Extraverted Thinkers are interested in organizing the

external world. They can give offense without meaning to because they focus on logical consequences instead of honoring the feelings of those involved.

To sum up: in addition to the eight players on your "team "(E, I, S, N, T, F, J and P), you can use your two perceiving functions (Sensing and iNtuition) and your two judging functions (Thinking and Feeling) in either Extravert (external world) or Introvert (what goes on inside you) mode. So you have four more players; twelve in all. More resources and more choices!

Conclusion:
The Art of Introversion

Yes, Introverts are different from Extraverts. Hallelu-jah! *I's* have some real natural advantages, as we've seen. For example: in depth of concentration; in focus; in thinking things through; and in being good listeners. (Remember, each of these is affected by the other aspects of personality as well.)

I's can and do excel at whatever they decide to do in the "real" world because they've thoroughly ana-lyzed and thought about it; before they take action, they play it through mentally to be sure everything will work out as desired.

Yes, Introverts may be a bit harder to get to know. But it is almost always worth the effort! They have great depth: still waters run deep.

Similarly, for every criticism leveled at Introverts (usually by Extraverts, who operate differently), there's a compensating strength which is the other side of the same coin. (That's true of Extraverts, also.)

Introverting— Only 25% of us are true Introverts; but 100% of us *do* some Introverting from time to time, every day.(Real Introverts are just better at it.)

But even Extraverts *can, do and must* Introvert, or they miss an important part of life and a vital skill. In order to get proper informational input and make good decisions, Extraverts must use their less-preferred Introvert side on a regular basis. Mental functions (as well as muscles) develop through exercise.

An Extravert friend said, "The message of your book is really, 'Hug an Introvert today!'" That's an Extravert response. First make sure the Introvert *wants* to be hugged, or even interrupted from his or her Introverting! Sometimes the greatest gift we can offer Introverts is privacy when they need it, quiet time— with the understanding that we're there when they want us to be. The message is, try to understand the differences between *I's* and *E's*, respect those differences, and appreciate the gifts of Introverts and the benefits of Introversion. And practice the skill of Introverting on a regular basis. It will improve your life.

About the Author...

Cheryl Card, consultant to companies and counselor to individuals, holds a BA from Cornell University and an MA from Johns-Hopkins and is a qualified administrator of the Myers-Briggs Type Indicator. A certified Human Potential Practitioner, she has been involved with People House of Denver since 1978 where she developed a passion for the introspective depth, beauty, power and potential for growth and recovery in group process work. After 20 years in business administration, Ms. Card now focuses on human resources and combines the human potential model, Gestalt therapy, and the psychology of type to help people find their true gifts. The mother of three, she believes it is particularly valuable for children and adolescents to understand and respect their own innate abilities and those of others.

Appendix

For more information on psychological type, see:

Barr, Lee & Norma, *The Leadership Equation.* Eakin Press, Austin, TX.

Ashley Brilliant & William D.G. Murray, *Give Your self the Unfair Advantage.* Type & Temperament, Inc., Gladwyne, PA.

Brownsword, Alan, *It Takes All Types.* HRM Press, San Anselmo, CA.

Delunas, Eve, *Survival Games Personalities Play.* Sunflower Ink, Carmel, CA.

Duniho, Terence, *Personalities at Risk.* Type & Temperament, Inc.,Gladwyne, PA.

Duniho, Terence, *Wellness vs. Neurotic Styles.* Type & Temperament, Inc., Gladwyne, PA.

Duniho, Terence, *Wholeness Lies Within.* Type & Temperament, Inc., Gladwyne, PA.

Duniho, Terence, *Your Shadow Side—The Fourth Function: Achilles Heel and Pearl of Great Price.* Type & Temperament, Inc., Gladwyne, PA.

Farris, Diane, *Type Tales for Children.* Consulting Psychologists Press, Inc. ,Palo Alto, CA.

Grant, Richard, *The I Ching.* Type & Temperament, Inc., Gladwyne, PA.

Grant, Richard, *Symbols of Recovery.* Type & Temperament, Inc, Gladwyne, PA.

Grant, Richard, *The Way of the Cross.* Type & Temperament, Inc. ,Gladwyne, PA.

Hirsh, Sandra Krebs, *Using the Myers-Briggs Type Indicator in Organizations.* Consulting Psychologists Press, Palo Alto, CA.

David Keirsey & Marilyn Bates, *Please Understand Me.* Prometheus Nemesis Book Company, Del Mar, CA.

Otto Kroeger & Janet Thuesen, *Type Talk.* Bantam Doubleday Dell (Delta, Tilden Press), NY.

Otto Kroeger & Janet Thuesen, *Type Talk at Work.* Bantam Doubleday Dell (Delta, Tilden Press), NY.

Murphy, Elizabeth, *The Developing Child: Using Jungian Type to Understand Children.* Consulting Psychologists Press, Palo Alto, CA.

Murray, William D.G., *And You Didn't Think You Had a Prayer.* Type &Temperament, Inc., Gladwyne, PA.

William D.G. Murray & Rosalie R. Murray, *Opposites.*Type & Temperament, Inc., Gladwyne, PA.

William D.G. Murray & Rosalie Murray, *When ENFP & INFJ Interact.* Type & Temperament, Inc., Gladwyne PA.

Isabel Briggs Myers & Peter B. Myers, *Gifts Differing.* Consulting Psychologists Press,Palo Alto, CA.

Page, Earle, *Looking at Type.* Center for Applications of Psychological Type, Gainesville, FL.

Sharp, Daryl, *Personality Types.* Inner City Books, Toronto, Ontario.

For more resources, request a catalog from:
Type & Temperament, Inc.
Box 200 Gladwyne, PA 19035-0200 USA
Tel. 1-(800) IHS-TYPE,
Outside US call (215) 527-2330
FAX (215) 527-1722.

My Notes